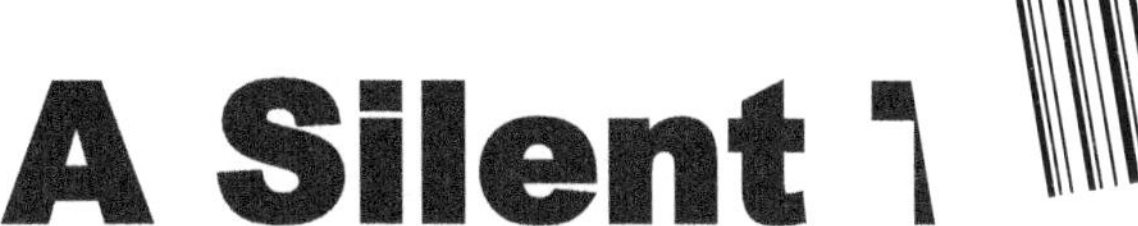

# Unlocking The Secrets to Reversing Fatty Liver Disease

Discover How to Regain Your Health and Prevent Chronic Conditions with Proven Diet, Lifestyle Changes, Warning Signs, Holistic Healing, and Effective Strategies

**By**

**George Leo**

# DEDICATION

To my family and friends, for their unwavering support and love. You've always stood by me through the journey of discovering the importance of liver health and the profound impact of diet and lifestyle. This book is a product of our shared passion for well-being, and I hope it serves as a guide to help many find better health and healing. To anyone struggling, remember: there is always hope, and change is possible. Let this be your first step towards transformation.

# ACKNOWLEDGMENTS

I would like to extend my deepest gratitude to the health professionals, researchers, and experts who contributed their invaluable knowledge to this book. Your insights have shaped its content and provided a strong foundation for understanding fatty liver disease. A special thank you to my readers—your stories of resilience and recovery inspired every page of this book. To my family, who supported me through the countless hours of research and writing, thank you for believing in me. This book is for all of you.

# TABLE OF CONTENTS

# INTRODUCTION

Imagine living with a condition that is slowly and silently eroding your health—yet, you have no idea it's happening. You wake up tired, struggle to focus, and wonder why your body just doesn't seem to respond the way it used to. Little do you know, your liver—one of the hardest-working organs in your body—is under siege. The culprit? Fatty liver disease. But here's the shocking part: you could have it right now without even knowing.

This isn't just another health scare—this is a silent epidemic sweeping through millions of people across the globe. Fatty liver disease doesn't have the loud, unmistakable symptoms that demand attention, but its consequences are real and potentially life-threatening. What's worse, most people have no clue they're on a path toward liver damage until it's too late. We call it a silent threat because it creeps up on you, quietly building in the background of your life, until one day, it's far too advanced to ignore.

But there's hope. This is not a diagnosis that means your life is over, nor is it something you have to live with indefinitely. Reversing fatty liver disease is possible, and it starts with you. This book is your roadmap to understanding what's happening inside your body, how to recognize the signs that you may already be struggling with fatty liver, and most importantly, how you can take control of your health today to reverse the damage and restore vitality to your life.

In the pages that follow, you'll uncover the truth behind this often misunderstood condition. You'll learn the real causes, the hidden triggers, and the strategies that work—strategies backed by science, not quick-fix gimmicks. You'll see how simple lifestyle changes, a targeted approach to nutrition, and a better understanding of your metabolic health can change the course of your liver's fate.

What you'll discover in this book will not only empower you to heal your liver but also give you the tools to prevent chronic diseases that could haunt you later in life—diseases like type 2 diabetes, heart disease, and even cancer. This is not just about treating one part of your body; it's about transforming your entire health and quality of life.

So, ask yourself: What if everything you thought you knew about liver disease was wrong? What if the key to reversing it lies in what you eat, how you live, and how you think? The journey you're about to embark on could be the most important of your life.

This isn't just a book. It's your first step toward a healthier, stronger, and more vibrant future. Get ready to unlock the secrets of your liver and reclaim the life you deserve.

# CHAPTER 1

## Understanding Fatty Liver Disease

Fatty liver disease—sounds harmless, doesn't it? Yet, it's one of the most insidious and dangerous conditions that millions of people unknowingly struggle with. It quietly takes root in your body, often without warning signs, until one day, it's too late to reverse the damage. Understanding what fatty liver disease is and how it operates within your body is the first step to taking control of your health.

At its core, fatty liver disease is the accumulation of excess fat in the liver cells. While it's easy to assume that this condition is linked only to heavy drinking, the truth is far more complex. There are two primary types of fatty liver disease: alcoholic fatty liver disease (AFLD) and non-alcoholic fatty liver disease (NAFLD).

Alcoholic fatty liver disease is the result of excessive alcohol consumption, which overwhelms the liver's ability to process and filter toxins. When alcohol is consumed in large amounts over time, it disrupts the liver's normal function, leading to fat accumulation in liver cells. However, non-alcoholic fatty liver disease (NAFLD), which is much more common, is not caused by alcohol. Instead, it is largely associated with factors such as obesity, poor diet, insulin resistance, and other metabolic conditions. NAFLD is particularly troubling because it can occur in people who don't drink at all, and it often goes unnoticed until more severe complications arise.

Fatty liver disease doesn't stay static—it progresses in stages. In its early form, it's known as simple fatty liver. Here, fat builds up in the liver, but there's little to no inflammation or damage to the liver cells. While simple fatty liver may seem mild, it can still lead to complications if left untreated. If the disease continues to progress, it can develop into non-alcoholic steatohepatitis (NASH). NASH is a more severe form, where the fat accumulation causes inflammation in the liver, leading to liver cell damage and scarring. This stage is dangerous because it increases the risk of cirrhosis, where the liver becomes severely scarred and its ability to function is compromised. In the worst-case scenario, fatty liver disease can progress to liver failure or even liver cancer, both of which are life-threatening.

One of the most frustrating aspects of fatty liver disease is its silent nature. In its early stages, it's often completely symptom-free. People with fatty liver disease may experience fatigue, feeling sluggish or tired for no apparent reason. This tiredness is often brushed off as a byproduct of stress, poor sleep, or just the demands of daily life. There may also be abdominal discomfort or a feeling of fullness in the upper right side of the abdomen. These symptoms are easily mistaken for something less severe, which is why many people go for years without knowing they have fatty liver disease. In some cases, people may notice skin issues—such as rashes or itchiness—but these are rarely linked directly to liver problems, leading to further confusion and misdiagnosis.

This is why it's crucial to act early. Fatty liver disease may not show symptoms until it reaches an advanced stage, but once the damage is done, it becomes much harder to reverse. If left unchecked, fatty liver disease can lead to liver cirrhosis, a condition where the liver becomes scarred and permanently damaged, making it unable to perform its vital functions. At this point, a liver transplant may be the only option. Worse still, the risk of developing liver cancer increases significantly as the liver deteriorates. These are not consequences that happen overnight—they are the result of years of untreated fatty liver disease, which is why early intervention is so crucial.

To truly understand why fatty liver disease is so dangerous, it's important to first grasp the role of the liver in our body. The liver is an incredibly resilient organ, capable of performing over 500 different functions. It's like the city's utilities system, managing everything from nutrient processing to waste removal. The liver's primary job is to filter out toxins, metabolize fats, and regulate blood sugar levels, keeping our body in balance. When the liver is overwhelmed by too much fat, it becomes less effective at carrying out these essential functions. This is why metabolism and detoxification are so closely linked to liver health. Without a healthy liver, your body struggles to manage energy, store nutrients, and fight off toxins, leading to a cascade of health problems that can affect your entire body.

Understanding the significance of the liver and how fatty liver disease can undermine its function is essential to grasping just how crucial it is to catch the disease early. With the right knowledge and the right approach, you can stop fatty liver disease in its tracks and take steps to heal your liver, restore its function, and protect your health. The journey to reversing fatty liver disease begins with recognizing the problem and understanding how to prevent it from progressing to more severe stages.

# CHAPTER 2

## Recognizing the Warning Signs

Fatty liver disease is often referred to as a silent condition, and for good reason. In the early stages, it rarely presents with noticeable symptoms, and even when symptoms do appear, they tend to be subtle—easily overlooked or attributed to other, less concerning causes. But as you read this, it's important to understand that these warning signs are your body's way of trying to communicate. While they may seem insignificant at first, ignoring them could allow fatty liver disease to silently progress to a more dangerous stage.

Fatigue is one of the most common and often underestimated early symptoms of fatty liver disease. Most of us are familiar with the feeling of tiredness, especially after a long day or stressful week. But when fatigue becomes constant—when you wake up feeling just as drained as when you went to bed—it might be your liver trying to tell you something. This relentless tiredness isn't always tied to a lack of sleep or emotional stress; it could be an indication that your liver is struggling to process the toxins and fats in your system.

Another common, but often dismissed, symptom is brain fog. It's that cloudy, sluggish feeling when you just can't focus, and simple tasks seem to take more effort than usual. You might find yourself forgetting things easily or feeling mentally drained, even though you've had a full night's rest. Many people chalk this up to stress or aging, but it could be a sign that the liver isn't detoxifying effectively, causing a build-up of waste that's affecting your cognitive function.

If you've also been experiencing mild abdominal discomfort, especially on the upper right side of your abdomen, this could be another subtle clue. The liver sits just beneath the ribcage, and as it becomes overwhelmed with fat, it can cause a feeling of fullness or tenderness. While this may not always translate into sharp pain, the discomfort is noticeable and could be exacerbated when you lie on your right side or press against that area.

Additionally, skin changes such as itchiness or rashes might also be signs that something's wrong. Fatty liver disease can cause the liver to lose its ability to process toxins effectively, leading to them building up in the body. As a result, this can manifest as skin irritation. Rashes, persistent itching, or even yellowing of the skin or eyes (called jaundice) are common symptoms of more advanced liver dysfunction, but they can start subtly as well.

While these subtle symptoms can easily be brushed off as signs of stress, aging, or a poor diet, they should never be ignored. If left unchecked, fatty liver disease can progress without noticeable symptoms until it reaches a much more dangerous stage. That's why it's crucial to recognize the red flags—the indicators that should make you stop and think, and possibly seek medical advice.

One of the most telling signs of fatty liver disease is elevated liver enzymes. These are substances that the liver produces in response to inflammation or damage. When the liver is stressed, such as with fatty liver disease, these enzymes can leak into the bloodstream. If your doctor performs a routine blood test and finds that your liver enzyme levels are higher than normal, it could be an indication that something isn't quite right.

Another important warning sign to be aware of is insulin resistance. Insulin is a hormone that helps regulate blood sugar levels. When your body becomes resistant to insulin, it forces your pancreas to produce more of it, which can lead to high blood sugar and, eventually, type 2 diabetes. Insulin resistance is closely linked to fatty liver disease because when the liver becomes overwhelmed with fat, it can't properly regulate blood sugar and lipids, exacerbating the condition. People who are overweight or have a high waist circumference are at a higher risk of developing insulin resistance, making it a crucial factor to monitor.

Metabolic syndrome, which includes a combination of risk factors like high blood pressure, high cholesterol, and high blood sugar, is another major red flag. If you've been diagnosed with any part of metabolic syndrome, it's time to talk to your doctor about fatty liver disease. Individuals with metabolic syndrome are significantly more likely to have fatty liver disease, and this combination of risk factors accelerates liver damage over time.

Lastly, belly fat and high cholesterol are strong indicators that your liver might be in trouble. Fat that accumulates around the abdomen—especially visceral fat, which surrounds the organs—can lead to inflammation and liver damage. This type of fat is particularly dangerous because it releases hormones and inflammatory chemicals that disrupt normal liver function. If you have high cholesterol, particularly elevated triglycerides, your liver's ability to process fat and maintain balance is compromised, making it more vulnerable to developing fatty liver disease.

So, when should you seek medical help? Fatty liver disease can progress for years without obvious signs, which is why it's vital to be proactive, especially if you have any of the risk factors we've discussed. The earlier fatty liver disease is diagnosed, the more effective the treatment will be. Many people wait until their condition has advanced to a more serious stage, only to find that significant damage has already occurred. That's why routine medical screening is essential—especially for those who have metabolic risk factors like obesity, type 2 diabetes, high blood pressure, or high cholesterol.

If you suspect you might have fatty liver disease, ask your doctor for a liver function test, which will measure enzymes that indicate liver stress or damage. A liver ultrasound can also provide visual evidence of fat accumulation in the liver, while a fibroscan—a non-invasive imaging technique—can assess the level of liver stiffness, which is a sign of scarring or fibrosis.

Taking these simple steps could be the difference between early intervention and irreversible liver damage. Don't wait until it's too late. Regular screenings, especially for high-risk individuals, can save your liver—and potentially your life.

# CHAPTER 3

## Common Myths About Fatty Liver Disease

When it comes to fatty liver disease, there's no shortage of myths and misconceptions that cloud people's understanding of this condition. These myths are dangerous because they prevent individuals from recognizing the risks they may face and can delay the vital steps needed for diagnosis and treatment. It's time to break through the noise and separate fact from fiction.

One of the most prevalent myths is that fatty liver disease is only caused by alcohol consumption. This misconception has persisted for decades, and it's understandable why. For years, the medical community focused on the relationship between alcohol and liver health, leading to the assumption that fatty liver disease could only occur in heavy drinkers. However, as research has advanced, we now know that alcohol is just one piece of the puzzle. While alcoholic fatty liver disease (AFLD) is indeed a concern for individuals who drink excessively, there is a far more common form of the disease that has nothing to do with alcohol. This condition is known as non-alcoholic fatty liver disease (NAFLD), and it affects millions of people around the world—many of whom don't drink alcohol at all.

In fact, non-alcoholic fatty liver disease (NAFLD) is far more widespread than alcoholic fatty liver disease, and it's linked to a variety of factors that go beyond alcohol consumption. NAFLD is primarily driven by insulin resistance, which is the body's inability to use insulin effectively. Insulin resistance is commonly associated with type 2 diabetes, obesity, and high cholesterol, but it can also develop in people who are not overtly overweight. This leads us to another misconception: that fatty liver disease is only a concern for overweight individuals.

It's easy to assume that only those who carry extra weight around their waist or hips would be at risk for fatty liver disease, but this is a dangerous oversimplification. The reality is that fatty liver disease can affect lean individuals as well, especially those with an underlying metabolic imbalance. These individuals may not appear overweight, but they could still be struggling with insulin resistance, a condition that makes it harder for the liver to process fat effectively. As a result, fat builds up in the liver, even in individuals with a healthy outward appearance. This form of fatty liver disease is often overlooked because many people don't associate liver issues with lean bodies.

So, why does this happen? The answer lies in our modern diet. We live in a world where refined carbohydrates, processed foods, and added sugars are prevalent in most people's daily intake. Even individuals who are lean might be consuming too much sugar and refined carbs, which wreak havoc on insulin sensitivity. The liver, trying to manage the overflow of sugar in the bloodstream, ends up converting it into fat, which accumulates in the liver over time. This accumulation can lead to NAFLD, and if left unchecked, can progress to more serious liver conditions such as non-alcoholic steatohepatitis (NASH), cirrhosis, and ultimately liver failure.

Now that we've debunked some common myths, it's important to understand what fatty liver disease really is and why it can affect individuals in ways we might not expect. Sugar and processed foods are the real culprits behind fatty liver disease, and they affect more than just people who are overweight. Even lean individuals can develop fatty liver disease if their diet is high in sugar, refined carbohydrates, and unhealthy fats. For example, someone who consumes a lot of sweetened beverages, fast food, and processed snacks could still be at risk, regardless of their weight.

The role of sugar in particular cannot be overstated. As the primary source of energy for the body, sugar plays a pivotal role in the development of fatty liver disease. When sugar is consumed in excess, the liver works overtime to process it, and the excess is converted into fat. This fat accumulates in the liver cells, causing the liver to become inflamed and overburdened. This leads to the development of non-alcoholic fatty liver disease (NAFLD), and eventually to more severe stages of liver damage.

This is why it's crucial to look beyond the surface level of obesity and lean body types when considering fatty liver disease. The disease can affect anyone, not just those who are overweight or drink excessively. The hidden risks are tied to lifestyle factors such as diet and insulin resistance, which often fly under the radar because they aren't immediately visible. A person can be lean, fit, and healthy-looking on the outside, but still struggle with fatty liver disease because of a diet that's too rich in sugar, refined grains, and processed foods. This is the silent nature of the disease—it doesn't discriminate based on appearance.

What you need to know is that fatty liver disease is not just about being overweight or drinking too much. It's about how your body handles what you eat and how it manages your metabolic processes. If you have insulin resistance, high cholesterol, or high blood sugar, you are at risk for fatty liver disease—regardless of how much you weigh or how healthy you think you are. The disease doesn't just affect obese individuals; it's a metabolic issue that can strike anyone, even those who appear healthy.

The good news is that fatty liver disease is reversible, especially in its early stages. By making simple lifestyle changes—adjusting your diet, becoming more physically active, and managing metabolic health—you can reduce fat accumulation in the liver, lower inflammation, and even restore liver function. It starts with understanding the true causes behind the disease and taking action before the damage becomes irreversible.

# CHAPTER 4

## The Link Between Sugar, Diet, and Fatty Liver Disease

When it comes to fatty liver disease, diet plays a pivotal role. It's not just about the fats you eat; it's about what else is fueling your body—specifically, sugar and refined carbohydrates. These elements are the silent instigators, slowly and steadily encouraging fat to accumulate in the liver, even in people who don't appear to be overweight. Understanding how these foods contribute to fatty liver disease is the first step toward taking control of your health and preventing the disease from spiraling out of control.

At the heart of the problem is sugar, specifically the overconsumption of refined sugar and refined carbohydrates. The body processes these sugars quickly, converting them into glucose that enters the bloodstream. As blood sugar levels rise, the liver is forced into overdrive, working to remove the excess sugar from circulation. Once the liver has dealt with the immediate glucose surge, it stores the excess energy in the form of fat, much of which gets deposited in liver cells. Over time, this fat accumulation begins to overwhelm the liver, leading to fatty liver disease.

But the liver doesn't just accumulate fat in isolation. When the liver is overloaded with fat, it starts to lose its ability to function properly. This is where insulin resistance comes into play. Insulin is a hormone that helps regulate blood sugar by allowing cells to absorb glucose for energy. But when you consume too much sugar or too many refined carbs, your body's cells become resistant to insulin. This means that insulin no longer does its job as effectively, leaving sugar circulating in the bloodstream at high levels. As a result, the liver is forced to produce even more fat to store the excess glucose, which leads to a vicious cycle of fat buildup and increasing insulin resistance.

The real problem, however, isn't just about the fat. It's about the sugar. While we've long known that fatty liver disease can result from excessive fat consumption, recent research has shown that sugar is the true culprit behind the liver's decline. To understand this, let's take a closer look at how sugar overload affects not just the liver, but the entire body—much like what we've seen in heart disease.

For years, we've been told that eating too much fat is the main cause of heart disease. The focus was on saturated fats and trans fats as the main villains, while sugar remained relatively unchallenged. However, more recent research has revealed that sugar—particularly in the form of refined carbohydrates and added sugars—is the primary driver behind heart disease and fatty liver disease. When we consume sugar, it not only leads to fat buildup in the liver but also increases inflammation in the body, a key factor in heart disease and other chronic conditions.

In particular, high-fructose corn syrup (HFCS) and refined grains are two of the biggest offenders. HFCS is a cheap, highly processed sweetener found in many processed foods, from sodas to snack bars. It is absorbed rapidly by the liver, where it is converted into fat. Unlike regular glucose, which can be processed by various cells in the body, fructose is almost entirely metabolized in the liver, making it especially harmful to liver health. This rapid conversion of sugar into fat makes the liver prone to developing fatty liver disease, and it can even increase the risk of more severe liver conditions like non-alcoholic steatohepatitis (NASH) and liver cirrhosis.

Similarly, refined grains, such as white bread, pasta, and rice, also play a significant role in fatty liver disease. These carbohydrates are stripped of their nutrients and fiber, making them more easily broken down into sugar, which floods the bloodstream. Much like high-fructose corn syrup, these refined grains contribute to an overload of sugar in the liver, leading to fat buildup and insulin resistance.

But it's not just about cutting sugar and refined carbs. Fats also play a role in liver health, and not all fats are created equal. Healthy fats, like those found in avocados, nuts, seeds, and olive oil, are essential for maintaining overall health. They help reduce inflammation, provide essential fatty acids for cellular repair, and support brain function. These healthy fats can even support liver function by improving insulin sensitivity and reducing fat accumulation in liver cells.

On the other hand, unhealthy fats, such as trans fats and saturated fats, have the opposite effect. Found in many processed and fried foods, these fats promote inflammation and disrupt the body's metabolic processes, leading to the development of fatty liver disease. When consumed in excess, trans fats and saturated fats contribute to increased fat storage in the liver and worsen insulin resistance, setting the stage for further liver damage.

Among the best fats to support liver health are omega-3 fatty acids, found in fatty fish like salmon, mackerel, and sardines. Omega-3s are known for their anti-inflammatory effects, which can help reduce the liver's fat load and improve insulin sensitivity. Studies have shown that omega-3s not only help lower fat accumulation in the liver but also help reduce the risk of fatty liver disease progression. If you don't eat enough fish, you can get omega-3s from plant-based sources like chia seeds, flaxseeds, and walnuts.

When we look at the impact of diet on fatty liver disease, it's clear that sugar, refined carbohydrates, and unhealthy fats are the real culprits. They overload the liver with fat, increase inflammation, and disrupt the body's metabolic processes. But by replacing these harmful elements with whole foods, healthy fats, and fiber-rich carbohydrates, you can support your liver and reduce the risk of fatty liver disease. The key is to focus on a diet that nourishes the liver and supports metabolic health, rather than relying on quick-fix solutions or fad diets.

As you move forward in your journey toward better liver health, it's important to remember that what you eat matters. Every meal is an opportunity to nourish your body, fuel your liver, and take control of your health. By making smart dietary choices and focusing on the foods that support liver function, you can reduce the risk of fatty liver disease and reclaim your vitality.

# CHAPTER 5

## The Importance of Liver Care Year-Round

When it comes to liver health, there's no magic bullet or quick fix. Too often, people are drawn to the promise of liver cleanses—detox diets or special kits that claim to rid the liver of toxins and restore its health in just a few days. These trendy solutions have captured the imagination of many, but the truth is that liver cleanses don't work.

The myth of the detox diet is built on the idea that our bodies need external help to clear out toxins. While it's true that the liver plays a crucial role in detoxification, it doesn't require cleanses or special supplements to function properly. In fact, the liver is one of the most resilient organs in the body, and it is fully equipped to handle the job of filtering toxins and processing fats, sugars, and proteins—year-round. What the liver needs isn't a one-time cleanse, but consistent, sustainable lifestyle changes that support its natural detoxification processes.

The myth of liver cleanses often leads people to believe that a few days of fasting or juicing can "reset" the liver, but this approach is ultimately ineffective and can even be harmful. Instead of focusing on a short-term fix, we should prioritize liver health as a continuous, daily commitment—one that requires steady, consistent effort over time. Long-term maintenance is the key to preserving liver function, ensuring that it continues to do its job efficiently without becoming overwhelmed by toxins or fat accumulation.

So, what does long-term liver care look like? It begins with the foundation of healthy lifestyle habits that support the liver on a daily basis. The first step is diet. As we've already discussed, sugar and refined carbohydrates can overload the liver, leading to fat buildup and, eventually, fatty liver disease. Eating a balanced, whole-foods diet rich in fiber, healthy fats, and lean proteins is essential for providing the liver with the nutrients it needs to function optimally. Reducing the intake of processed foods, sugars, and unhealthy fats is a critical part of keeping the liver healthy.

But diet alone is not enough. The liver also benefits from hydration. Water plays a pivotal role in helping the liver flush out toxins. When you're dehydrated, your liver's ability to detoxify your body becomes compromised. Drinking plenty of water throughout the day ensures that the liver has what it needs to keep toxins flowing out of the system, preventing the buildup of harmful substances.

In addition to hydration, exercise is another cornerstone of long-term liver care. Regular physical activity not only helps reduce fat accumulation in the liver but also improves insulin sensitivity, which is crucial for preventing or reversing fatty liver disease. Exercise helps burn off excess fat, maintain a healthy weight, and improve circulation—all of which contribute to better liver function. Whether it's walking, running, yoga, or strength training, being active on a consistent basis supports the liver and metabolic health as a whole.

Another often-overlooked aspect of liver maintenance is toxin reduction. While the liver is designed to detoxify the body, it can become overloaded when we're constantly exposed to environmental toxins, chemicals, and pollutants. Reducing exposure to harmful substances—such as household cleaners, pesticides, and airborne pollutants—helps alleviate the strain on the liver. Similarly, avoiding excessive alcohol consumption and reducing your exposure to smoking or secondhand smoke can protect the liver from unnecessary damage. Supporting the liver means making conscious choices to minimize the toxin load on the body.

It's also essential to remember that liver care is a long-term commitment. Just like any aspect of health, the key to maintaining a strong, healthy liver is consistency. There's no quick fix, no single cleanse or supplement that can replace the daily habits that protect the liver. The idea that one can "reset" the liver with a quick detox is an illusion. What truly benefits the liver is daily care, gradual improvements, and sustainable changes that add up over time.

Ultimately, the goal is to make liver-friendly habits a permanent part of your lifestyle. Think of it this way: if you were to care for a valuable piece of equipment, you wouldn't just focus on fixing it once in a while—you would take care of it regularly, with ongoing attention to its needs. Your liver is no different. It is an incredibly resilient organ, capable of regenerating itself and handling the demands you place on it. But just like any other system in the body, it thrives on consistent, mindful care. The best way to support your liver and ensure its health for years to come is through everyday lifestyle choices that prioritize nutrition, hydration, movement, and toxin reduction.

# CHAPTER 6

## Alcohol and Its Impact on Liver Health

When it comes to liver health, alcohol is often viewed through a complicated lens. We've all heard the debate: is moderate drinking really as harmful as we think? Can a glass of wine a day really hurt your liver? The reality is that alcohol, even in small quantities, can place a significant strain on the liver, especially over time.

### Alcohol's Role in Liver Stress

The liver is responsible for processing and metabolizing alcohol in the body. When you consume alcohol, the liver breaks it down, but this process comes with a cost. Alcohol is viewed by the liver as a toxin—something that needs to be neutralized and removed from the body. For the liver, this means shifting its focus from other vital tasks to detoxifying the alcohol. The more alcohol you consume, the harder your liver has to work.

Even in small amounts, alcohol can be stressful to the liver. The liver breaks down alcohol into acetaldehyde, a substance that is toxic to liver cells. While the liver is highly resilient and can handle some level of alcohol, excessive drinking over time can lead to a buildup of fat, inflammation, and ultimately liver damage. Fatty liver disease and cirrhosis are common outcomes for those who regularly consume excessive alcohol, and in many cases, people may not even feel the symptoms until the liver is already severely compromised.

However, it's not just about the quantity of alcohol you drink, but also the regularity. Chronic alcohol consumption—even in what is often considered "moderate" amounts—can gradually wear down the liver, making it more susceptible to developing fatty liver disease and other serious conditions. This is why even seemingly healthy habits, like having a glass of wine with dinner every night, can eventually have a damaging effect on liver health. The liver doesn't get a break from its detoxifying duties, and over time, the cumulative stress can be overwhelming.

## Defining Moderate Drinking

There's been a long-standing belief that moderate alcohol consumption doesn't pose a significant risk to liver health. But what exactly does "moderate" mean, and is it truly safe for the liver?

The CDC and other health organizations define moderate drinking as up to one drink per day for women and up to two drinks per day for men. A "drink" is typically defined as:

- **One 12-ounce beer** (5% alcohol)

- **One 5-ounce glass of wine** (12% alcohol)
- **One 1.5-ounce shot of distilled spirits** (40% alcohol)

While these guidelines are intended to provide some clarity, they don't take into account the unique impact alcohol can have on individuals with existing health conditions, such as fatty liver disease or metabolic syndrome. For people with fatty liver disease, even small amounts of alcohol can exacerbate the condition. Drinking alcohol, even within moderate limits, can worsen liver inflammation and hinder the liver's ability to process fat, potentially leading to the progression from simple fatty liver to non-alcoholic steatohepatitis (NASH) and even cirrhosis.

The truth is that moderate drinking can still have negative effects on liver health, especially for those already at risk for fatty liver disease. So, while the occasional glass of wine may not immediately cause harm, for those with existing liver issues, the safest approach is to either minimize or eliminate alcohol entirely.

### The Dangers of Alcohol Consumption for Individuals with Fatty Liver Disease

For individuals already dealing with fatty liver disease, alcohol consumption poses significant dangers. Even small amounts of alcohol can accelerate the progression of fatty liver disease, potentially leading to liver fibrosis, cirrhosis, and even liver cancer. Alcohol adds additional toxicity to the liver, causing inflammation and compounding the fat buildup that characterizes NAFLD (non-alcoholic fatty liver disease).

In cases where individuals already have non-alcoholic fatty liver disease (NAFLD), drinking alcohol—no matter how moderate—can significantly increase the liver's workload, speeding up the progression of the disease and making it harder for the liver to regenerate and repair itself. For those in the early stages of fatty liver disease, eliminating alcohol is one of the most effective ways to reduce liver stress and help the body begin healing. Continuing to drink, even occasionally, can prevent the liver from getting the necessary rest and support it needs to recover and reduce fat accumulation.

For those with advanced liver damage, such as cirrhosis, alcohol consumption can be fatal. Cirrhosis weakens the liver's ability to function and dramatically increases the risk of complications like liver failure and liver cancer. The body's ability to metabolize alcohol becomes severely compromised, leading to severe liver dysfunction. It's essential for those with advanced liver disease to understand the gravity of alcohol consumption and consider complete abstinence to manage their condition effectively.

Alternatives to Alcohol

While the risks of alcohol consumption are clear, that doesn't mean you have to live without alternatives that allow you to still enjoy a satisfying drink. Fortunately, there is a growing range of non-alcoholic options that can support your liver health while satisfying your cravings for a flavorful beverage.

Non-alcoholic beverages, such as sparkling water, herbal teas, and fresh juices, can be refreshing and hydrating alternatives to alcohol. For those who miss the experience of having a drink in hand, there are now non-alcoholic wines, beers, and spirits available on the market. These beverages provide the taste and sensation of alcohol without the harmful effects on the liver. Additionally, many of these non-alcoholic drinks are made with natural ingredients, making them a healthier choice overall.

The benefits of reducing or eliminating alcohol are profound. Not only does this decision protect your liver, but it can also improve your sleep quality, mental clarity, and overall well-being. By switching to non-alcoholic alternatives, you give your liver the best chance to heal and maintain its crucial functions without the added stress of alcohol processing.

# CHAPTER 7

## Metabolic Health and Fatty Liver Disease

When we talk about fatty liver disease, it's impossible to ignore the intricate connection between metabolic health and liver function. In fact, one of the main drivers of non-alcoholic fatty liver disease (NAFLD) is metabolic dysfunction, which includes a combination of risk factors like obesity, type 2 diabetes, high blood pressure, and abnormal cholesterol levels. This is why metabolic syndrome is often referred to as a key precursor to fatty liver disease—people with metabolic syndrome are at a much higher risk of developing liver issues that can ultimately lead to cirrhosis or liver failure if not managed properly.

## Understanding Metabolic Syndrome

Metabolic syndrome is a term used to describe a cluster of conditions that increase your risk of heart disease, stroke, and type 2 diabetes. These conditions often go hand-in-hand with fatty liver disease, as they share many common risk factors. If you are obese or have excess abdominal fat, insulin resistance, high blood pressure, or elevated blood sugar and cholesterol, you're more likely to develop fatty liver disease. It's not just about weight, but where the weight is stored—specifically, fat around the belly (visceral fat), which has a much stronger association with liver disease than fat stored in other parts of the body.

The connection is clear: obesity, insulin resistance, and high cholesterol all put extra strain on the liver. Excess fat in the liver leads to inflammation, which can make insulin resistance worse, further contributing to the cycle. When the liver can no longer properly process fats or manage blood sugar, it accumulates more fat, worsening the condition and leading to fatty liver disease.

One of the key signs that someone may be at risk for fatty liver disease is their waist circumference. Studies have shown that individuals with excess fat around their waist are more likely to have fatty liver disease, even if they are not technically overweight by the typical BMI (body mass index) standards. This is because visceral fat, the fat that surrounds internal organs like the liver, is particularly harmful and more likely to contribute to liver fat buildup.

## The Four Metabolic Types

In order to understand your risk of developing fatty liver disease, it's important to recognize that there isn't a one-size-fits-all approach. People's metabolisms differ, and these differences are often categorized into four distinct metabolic types: Preventer, Fine-Tuner, Recalibrator, and Regenerator. These types help to identify how your body processes food and stores fat, as well as the risks you may face when it comes to liver health.

- The Preventer: This person is typically lean and metabolically healthy. They don't have issues with insulin resistance or metabolic dysfunction. Their risk for fatty liver disease is low, and they maintain a healthy weight with good lifestyle habits.
- The Fine-Tuner: These individuals are healthy in many ways, but they carry excess fat around their belly. While their metabolic markers like blood sugar and cholesterol levels are mostly normal, they have a higher risk of developing fatty liver disease due to their central obesity. These individuals can significantly reduce their risk by losing excess weight and making healthier lifestyle choices.

- The Recalibrator: The recalibrator is someone who is unhealthy but lean—they may not have visible abdominal fat, but their metabolic markers, such as elevated blood sugar, insulin resistance, or high cholesterol, indicate a higher risk for liver disease. Even if they are not overweight, this group needs to focus on improving their metabolic health through dietary and lifestyle adjustments to reduce their risk of fatty liver disease.
- The Regenerator: This group represents those who are unhealthy and unlean. These individuals are at the highest risk for fatty liver disease and its complications. They carry excess fat around their belly and have metabolic dysfunction (such as insulin resistance, high cholesterol, and high blood pressure). However, they also have the highest potential for improvement through lifestyle changes—losing weight, improving insulin sensitivity, and reducing inflammation can make a significant difference in their liver health.

Understanding which metabolic type you belong to is an essential part of assessing your risk for fatty liver disease. Each metabolic type has its own set of challenges and opportunities for improvement. By recognizing your type, you can take proactive steps to manage your metabolic health and protect your liver.

**Managing Your Metabolic Health**

The key to reversing or preventing fatty liver disease lies in managing metabolic health effectively. This involves a combination of dietary changes, exercise, and stress management to improve insulin sensitivity, reduce inflammation, and achieve metabolic balance.

1. Improving Insulin Sensitivity: One of the most important steps in managing metabolic health is improving how your body responds to insulin. When you become insulin resistant, the body struggles to process glucose, which leads to fat accumulation in the liver. A diet rich in whole foods, fiber, and healthy fats, and low in processed

sugars and refined carbohydrates, can improve insulin sensitivity. Exercise, particularly strength training and aerobic activity, can also enhance insulin sensitivity, helping the liver and other organs function more efficiently.

2. Reducing Inflammation: Chronic inflammation is a hallmark of metabolic dysfunction and fatty liver disease. Anti-inflammatory foods, such as omega-3 fatty acids from fish and flaxseeds, green leafy vegetables, and turmeric, can help reduce inflammation in the body. Avoiding pro-inflammatory foods like trans fats and processed sugars will also help reduce the strain on the liver.
3. Achieving Metabolic Balance: It's important to address all aspects of metabolic health, not just liver health. By losing excess weight, particularly visceral fat, improving cholesterol levels, and managing blood sugar, you reduce your risk of fatty liver disease and other chronic health conditions. Finding balance means adopting a

holistic approach to health, incorporating regular exercise, a balanced diet, and stress management practices such as yoga, meditation, or adequate sleep.

Taking action today to manage your metabolic health is not just about avoiding fatty liver disease—it's about protecting your body from a cascade of other health issues, including heart disease, stroke, and type 2 diabetes. Through small but consistent changes in your daily habits, you can begin to reclaim your health, improve liver function, and reduce your overall risk for metabolic diseases.

# CHAPTER 8

## Gut Health and the Liver Connection

When most people think of the liver, they picture an organ devoted to processing fats and detoxifying the body. While this is true, there is another crucial relationship that often goes overlooked—the connection between the liver and the gut microbiome. Over the past few years, researchers have discovered that the gut microbiome, the trillions of bacteria living in our digestive system, plays a significant role in the health of our liver. It turns out, the gut is more than just a digestive powerhouse—it is a central player in metabolic health and the liver's ability to function optimally.

### The Microbiome's Impact on the Liver

The gut microbiome is not a passive system; it is highly active, influencing many aspects of our body's health. The gut bacteria play a critical role in metabolizing nutrients, producing vitamins, and supporting the immune system. But beyond these functions, the microbiome directly impacts liver health by influencing how the liver processes fats, sugars, and other nutrients. The gut and liver are in constant communication, often referred to as the gut-liver axis.

When the gut microbiome is in balance, it helps the liver perform its crucial functions, including detoxification, fat metabolism, and protein synthesis. However, when the gut microbiome becomes disrupted, the liver is often the first organ to suffer. Dysbiosis, a condition where harmful bacteria outnumber beneficial ones, can lead to a cascade of metabolic problems, including fatty liver disease. The liver, under constant strain from the poor signals it receives from an imbalanced microbiome, begins to accumulate fat and develop inflammation, setting the stage for liver disease.

This gut-liver connection is especially important when considering how metabolic diseases like obesity, insulin resistance, and type 2 diabetes interact with fatty liver disease. Studies show that an unhealthy gut microbiome can directly contribute to the development of insulin resistance, which, in turn, can lead to fatty liver disease. So, maintaining a healthy gut is not just important for digestion, but essential for the overall health of your liver.

## Disrupting the Gut Microbiome

Many modern-day lifestyle factors can disrupt the balance of our gut microbiome, leading to negative effects on the liver. Sugar, processed foods, and alcohol are some of the biggest offenders when it comes to gut health.

Sugar and refined carbohydrates are known to fuel the growth of harmful bacteria in the gut, creating an imbalance that promotes inflammation. These foods cause blood sugar spikes, leading to insulin resistance, which, as we've seen, can directly contribute to fatty liver disease. Not only does excess sugar negatively affect the microbiome, but it also forces the liver to process and store it as fat, contributing to liver fat accumulation and further metabolic dysfunction.

Processed foods are another major disruptor. These foods often contain artificial additives, preservatives, and trans fats that can damage the lining of the gut and promote the overgrowth of harmful bacteria. This damage leads to a condition called leaky gut, where the gut lining becomes permeable and allows toxins and bacteria to leak into the bloodstream. This triggers inflammation, which then extends to the liver, worsening the symptoms of fatty liver disease and making it more difficult for the liver to detoxify effectively.

Alcohol has long been known for its harmful effects on the liver, but its impact on the gut is just as significant. Chronic alcohol consumption disrupts the balance of the microbiome, leading to an overgrowth of pathogenic bacteria. These harmful bacteria then produce toxins that can reach the liver, exacerbating liver damage and inflammation. Alcohol also contributes to leaky gut, allowing harmful substances to enter the bloodstream, further straining the liver's detoxification processes.

Together, these factors create a perfect storm for liver health, setting the stage for the development of fatty liver disease and other chronic health issues.

## Supporting a Healthy Gut for Liver Health

Given the crucial link between the gut and liver, it is essential to support a healthy gut microbiome to maintain liver function. A balanced microbiome not only promotes optimal liver health, but also helps regulate metabolic processes that are critical for detoxification, fat metabolism, and insulin sensitivity. The key to achieving and maintaining a healthy gut lies in the consumption of prebiotics, probiotics, and fiber—all of which are vital for nurturing the beneficial bacteria in the gut.

Prebiotics are food sources that help nourish the healthy bacteria in your gut. These include fiber-rich foods, such as whole grains, legumes, onions, garlic, and bananas. Prebiotics support the growth of beneficial bacteria, creating an environment where good microbes thrive and harmful bacteria are kept in check. When the gut is properly nourished with prebiotics, the liver benefits from a healthier, more efficient microbiome.

Probiotics, on the other hand, are live beneficial bacteria that can be consumed through fermented foods like yogurt, kefir, sauerkraut, and kimchi. Probiotics help replenish and restore the balance of beneficial bacteria in the gut. These microorganisms are essential for breaking down food, producing vital nutrients, and regulating the immune system. Probiotics also play a role in reducing inflammation, which is a key factor in both insulin resistance and fatty liver disease.

In addition to prebiotics and probiotics, fiber is one of the most important components of a gut-friendly diet. High-fiber foods, such as vegetables, fruits, legumes, and whole grains, provide fuel for healthy gut bacteria. Fiber helps regulate bowel movements, improve gut health, and reduce inflammation. It also assists in the detoxification process, helping the liver flush out toxins more efficiently.

Some specific foods that promote a balanced microbiome and support liver health include:

- Leafy greens, such as spinach and kale, which are rich in antioxidants and fiber.
- Berries, which are packed with antioxidants and help reduce inflammation.

- Fermented foods, such as kimchi, sauerkraut, and miso, which provide a natural source of probiotics.
- Omega-3 rich foods, such as salmon, chia seeds, and flaxseeds, which support healthy liver function and reduce inflammation.
- Garlic and onions, which are excellent sources of prebiotics.

By focusing on a gut-friendly diet, you can support your liver and reduce the risk of fatty liver disease. It's not just about reducing the bad foods like sugar and processed items; it's equally about adding the right foods that nourish the gut and allow the liver to function optimally.

# CHAPTER 9

## Foods That Heal the Liver

The liver is a remarkable organ. It has the power to regenerate, filter toxins, and keep our bodies in balance. But like any other system in the body, it requires the right fuel to function optimally. And while many people think of liver health only in terms of avoiding alcohol or treating disease with medication, the truth is that food plays a pivotal role in supporting liver function. What we eat—or more importantly, what we don't eat—can either promote liver damage or help heal and protect it. If you're looking to restore your liver health, there are plenty of foods that can support its recovery and even reverse damage over time.

## Liver-Friendly Foods

There are certain foods that stand out when it comes to liver health. They are packed with nutrients that promote detoxification, reduce inflammation, and protect the liver from oxidative stress. Here's a breakdown of 12 powerful foods that can nourish your liver and help it heal:

- Coffee: Surprisingly, coffee is one of the most liver-friendly beverages you can drink. It's loaded with antioxidants and has been shown to reduce the risk of liver disease, including non-alcoholic fatty liver disease (NAFLD). Studies suggest that coffee helps lower liver enzymes, which is an important marker for liver function. It also helps reduce inflammation and prevent the development of liver fibrosis (scarring). Drinking coffee regularly, particularly without added sugars and creamers, supports liver health in significant ways.

- Berries: Berries, such as blueberries, blackberries, and raspberries, are packed with antioxidants that help reduce liver inflammation. These antioxidants, especially flavonoids and polyphenols, neutralize free radicals that can damage liver cells. They also play a role in reducing oxidative stress, a condition that accelerates liver damage and contributes to the progression of fatty liver disease.
- Kiwi: This small, vibrant fruit is a powerhouse of nutrients, including vitamin C, fiber, and antioxidants. Kiwi has been shown to help reduce oxidative stress in the liver and improve overall liver function. It's also a great source of prebiotics, which support the growth of healthy bacteria in the gut, indirectly benefiting the liver by improving digestion and reducing inflammation.
- Dark Chocolate: It may come as a pleasant surprise, but dark chocolate, particularly varieties with 70% cocoa or higher, is a great food for liver

health. It's rich in flavonoids, which have anti-inflammatory properties and help protect the liver from damage. Moderate consumption of dark chocolate has been linked to improved liver function and reduced liver fat accumulation.

- Edamame: These young soybeans are rich in isoflavones, which are plant compounds that help reduce liver inflammation. They are also a good source of protein and fiber, both of which support liver detoxification. The fiber content in edamame aids digestion and helps lower cholesterol, which is critical for maintaining liver health.
- Fatty Fish: Salmon, mackerel, and sardines are some of the best sources of omega-3 fatty acids, which are essential for liver health. Omega-3s reduce liver fat and inflammation, which are common issues in fatty liver disease. These healthy fats also help balance blood lipids and improve insulin sensitivity, reducing the risk of metabolic diseases that can harm the liver.

- Leafy Greens: Vegetables like spinach, kale, and arugula are rich in chlorophyll, which helps the liver detoxify by removing harmful chemicals from the bloodstream. These greens are also high in fiber, which supports digestion and liver function. The anti-inflammatory compounds in leafy greens can help reduce liver inflammation, particularly in conditions like NAFLD.
- Turmeric: Known for its bright yellow color, turmeric contains curcumin, a potent antioxidant with powerful anti-inflammatory properties. Curcumin has been shown to reduce liver damage and help heal liver tissue. It also supports the liver in detoxifying the body and preventing fat accumulation.
- Garlic: This kitchen staple has more to offer than just flavor. Garlic contains allicin, a compound that helps reduce inflammation and oxidative stress in the liver. It also helps improve liver function by stimulating the production of liver

enzymes that detoxify harmful substances from the body.

- Olive Oil: High-quality extra virgin olive oil is rich in monounsaturated fats and antioxidants, making it a great choice for liver health. It helps reduce liver fat and inflammation while improving insulin sensitivity. The healthy fats in olive oil also help to lower bad cholesterol, supporting both liver and heart health.
- Beets: Beets are a great source of betaine, a compound that supports liver detoxification by helping to flush out toxins. They also contain high levels of fiber, which promotes digestion and overall gut health. The antioxidants in beets help reduce inflammation, improving liver health over time.
- Avocado: Rich in healthy fats, fiber, and antioxidants, avocados help protect liver cells from damage. Studies have shown that avocados may even help reduce liver fat and improve liver

function in individuals with fatty liver disease. The glutathione in avocados also plays a key role in detoxifying the liver.

**The Power of Fiber**

When it comes to liver health, fiber is one of the most powerful nutrients you can consume. Fiber helps support the liver's detoxification processes, ensuring that harmful toxins are flushed from the body rather than accumulating in the liver. Fiber also helps lower cholesterol levels and stabilize blood sugar, both of which are critical for preventing fatty liver disease. Foods like legumes, whole grains, fruits, and vegetables are all excellent sources of fiber that nourish the liver and promote overall metabolic health.

Fiber-rich foods also improve gut health, which is critical for liver function. A healthy gut microbiome helps regulate insulin sensitivity, reduces inflammation, and enhances nutrient absorption. All of these factors contribute to a healthier liver and reduced risk of fatty liver disease.

## Antioxidants and Anti-Inflammatory Foods

Antioxidants are compounds that help neutralize free radicals—unstable molecules that can damage liver cells and contribute to oxidative stress. Foods high in antioxidants, such as berries, dark chocolate, leafy greens, and turmeric, can help protect the liver from damage and prevent the progression of liver disease.

In addition to antioxidants, anti-inflammatory foods are also essential for liver health. Chronic inflammation is a key driver of liver disease, and reducing it is crucial for preventing further damage. Foods rich in omega-3 fatty acids, such as fatty fish and olive oil, have strong anti-inflammatory effects, as do turmeric and garlic.

By incorporating a variety of antioxidant-rich and anti-inflammatory foods into your diet, you can significantly improve liver function and reduce the risk of fatty liver disease and other chronic conditions.

## Building a Liver-Supportive Diet

Creating a liver-supportive diet is not about following rigid rules or cutting out entire food groups. It's about focusing on whole, nutrient-dense foods that nourish the liver and support its function. To start, aim to incorporate more fiber-rich foods like fruits, vegetables, and whole grains into your meals. Add healthy fats from avocados, olive oil, and fatty fish to your diet to promote anti-inflammatory and detoxifying benefits. And don't forget to enjoy the liver-healing benefits of coffee, berries, and dark chocolate in moderation.

Meal planning for liver health doesn't have to be complicated. Focus on balance and variety, and aim to include foods from each of the liver-friendly categories mentioned above. For example, a typical day could include a green smoothie with spinach, kiwi, and flaxseeds for breakfast; a salmon salad with olive oil and mixed greens for lunch; and grilled chicken with roasted beets and avocado for dinner. Incorporate nuts, seeds, and berries as snacks throughout the day to ensure you're getting the antioxidants and healthy fats your liver needs.

# CHAPTER 10

## The Role of Exercise in Liver Health

When we think about improving our health, the mind often jumps to diet and medications. But there is one powerful tool that can significantly enhance liver health—exercise. It is well-known that physical activity offers numerous benefits for the body, from boosting heart health to improving mental well-being. But what many people don't realize is just how essential exercise is for maintaining and improving liver function. In fact, regular physical activity is one of the most effective ways to combat fatty liver disease and support the liver's detoxification process.

### Why Exercise is Key for Fatty Liver Disease

The liver plays a critical role in metabolism, breaking down fats, carbohydrates, and proteins, as well as detoxifying harmful substances from the blood. When fatty liver disease develops, the liver becomes overwhelmed with excess fat, leading to fat accumulation and inflammation. This can eventually progress to non-alcoholic steatohepatitis (NASH) or even cirrhosis, causing permanent damage.

Exercise, however, can play a pivotal role in reversing fatty liver disease. Regular physical activity helps reduce fat in the liver, improve insulin sensitivity, and reduce inflammation. When we engage in physical activity, our muscles use energy, which in turn helps the body burn fat more efficiently. This reduction in fat storage—especially in the liver—can significantly improve liver health and even reverse early-stage fatty liver disease.

One of the key ways that exercise helps the liver is by improving insulin sensitivity. When the body becomes resistant to insulin, the liver starts storing excess fat as a protective measure, leading to fatty liver disease. Exercise, particularly aerobic or cardiovascular exercises, helps the body utilize insulin more effectively, reducing the liver's need to store fat. This not only helps prevent further fat buildup but also encourages the liver to start burning fat rather than storing it.

## Types of Exercise That Benefit the Liver

Not all exercise is created equal when it comes to liver health. However, a combination of cardiovascular exercise, strength training, and flexibility exercises can provide optimal benefits for the liver.

- Cardiovascular Exercise: Activities such as walking, jogging, swimming, and cycling are excellent for improving liver health. These exercises elevate the heart rate, increase blood circulation, and help the body burn fat.

Cardiovascular exercises are particularly effective at reducing liver fat and improving insulin sensitivity. A study published in the Journal of Hepatology found that moderate-intensity aerobic exercise significantly reduced liver fat in people with non-alcoholic fatty liver disease (NAFLD).

- Strength Training: Lifting weights or engaging in resistance training helps to build muscle mass. More muscle mass improves overall metabolism, which in turn helps to burn fat more efficiently. Strength training also plays a role in improving insulin sensitivity and balancing blood sugar levels, both of which are essential for managing fatty liver disease. Studies have shown that strength training, in combination with cardiovascular exercise, is highly effective at reducing liver fat and improving liver function.
- Flexibility Exercises: While yoga, stretching, and Pilates may not directly target fat loss, they play an important role in maintaining overall health.

Flexibility exercises help reduce stress and improve circulation, both of which can support liver health. Yoga has also been shown to reduce inflammation and improve insulin sensitivity, making it an excellent complementary practice for those looking to improve liver health.

Incorporating these three types of exercises—cardiovascular, strength training, and flexibility exercises—into your routine can provide comprehensive benefits for liver function. The combination of fat-burning, muscle-building, and stress-reducing exercises is ideal for managing and even reversing fatty liver disease.

### Creating an Exercise Routine

The key to improving liver health through exercise is consistency. It's not about pushing yourself to extreme limits or committing to hours of intense workouts. The goal is to incorporate regular movement into your daily routine and gradually increase intensity over time.

Starting with small, manageable goals is the best approach. For example, aim for 30 minutes of moderate-intensity cardiovascular exercise five days a week. This could be something as simple as going for a brisk walk or bike ride. If you're new to exercise, start slow and gradually build up your stamina. Begin with 10 to 15-minute sessions and slowly increase the duration as you become more comfortable.

Strength training can be done two to three times per week, using bodyweight exercises (such as squats, lunges, and push-ups) or light weights. As you progress, you can increase the intensity by adding more weight or doing more challenging exercises. A good goal is to focus on full-body strength rather than targeting individual muscles. This helps to increase overall muscle mass, which boosts metabolism and supports liver health.

Flexibility exercises, such as yoga or stretching, can be practiced daily, even if only for a few minutes. These exercises will help improve flexibility, reduce tension, and promote relaxation. If you're short on time, try starting or ending your day with a simple 10-minute yoga routine.

Remember that the key to success is consistency. Make exercise a regular part of your routine, and don't get discouraged if you miss a day or two. The more consistent you are, the better the results will be. And as you progress, you'll notice improvements in your energy levels, overall health, and liver function.

## The Importance of Consistency Over Time

When it comes to liver health and exercise, consistency is crucial. While a single workout can help boost metabolism and burn fat, the true benefits of exercise on liver health come when physical activity becomes a part of your regular lifestyle. In order to see lasting improvements in liver function, it's important to stick with your exercise routine over time.

One of the most powerful aspects of regular exercise is its ability to create lasting changes in the body. With time, your body will become more efficient at burning fat, regulating blood sugar, and processing nutrients. This results in a healthier liver, a more balanced metabolism, and reduced inflammation—all of which are essential for managing fatty liver disease.

Ultimately, liver health is about sustainability. Exercise should not be seen as a temporary fix, but rather a lifelong commitment to supporting your liver and overall well-being. The changes you make today—whether it's going for a walk, lifting weights, or practicing yoga—will pay off in the long run by improving your liver health and reducing the risk of future liver disease.

# CHAPTER 11

## Reversing Fatty Liver Disease

The liver is a remarkable organ, often referred to as the body's "detox powerhouse." Its ability to regenerate is nothing short of extraordinary. The liver can heal itself when given the proper care and support, making it one of the few organs capable of reversing damage if the right steps are taken early. For those struggling with fatty liver disease, this offers a beacon of hope: with lifestyle changes, dietary adjustments, and consistent effort, the liver can regenerate, and the progression of fatty liver disease can be reversed, or at least mitigated.

### The Liver's Regenerative Power

One of the most fascinating aspects of the liver is its regenerative power. Unlike many organs in the body, the liver has the remarkable ability to heal itself. Even after injury or damage, the liver can regenerate healthy tissue, as long as the damage isn't too severe. This regenerative ability is why many liver conditions, including fatty liver disease, can often be managed effectively when detected early. The liver, when properly supported, can regenerate healthy tissue and regain full function.

However, this regenerative power is not infinite. The liver's ability to repair itself diminishes when the damage becomes too severe, as in the case of cirrhosis or advanced stages of liver disease. This is why early intervention is crucial. If fatty liver disease is identified early, lifestyle changes such as diet modification, exercise, and regular screenings can help stop the progression of the disease and allow the liver to begin healing itself.

**Strategies for Reversing Early-Stage Fatty Liver**

For those in the early stages of fatty liver disease, there is a clear path forward. The key to reversing early-stage fatty liver disease lies in lifestyle changes, primarily through diet, exercise, and regular medical screenings.

- Diet: A healthy, balanced diet is paramount. Cutting out excess sugars, refined carbohydrates, and processed foods is crucial in reducing fat accumulation in the liver. Emphasizing a diet rich in whole foods, fiber, and healthy fats can help reduce liver fat and promote liver function. Foods such as berries, leafy greens, healthy oils (like olive oil), omega-3 rich fish, and lean proteins should be staples in the diet. Reducing processed sugars and replacing refined carbohydrates with whole grains and high-fiber vegetables will significantly help reduce liver fat. Additionally, staying hydrated with water and avoiding excess alcohol consumption are fundamental to supporting liver regeneration.
- Exercise: Regular physical activity is just as crucial in reversing fatty liver disease as diet. Aerobic exercises, like walking, cycling, and swimming, can

help burn fat stored in the liver, improving its function and reducing fat accumulation. Strength training also plays a role by boosting metabolism and helping the body burn fat more efficiently. Exercise has the added benefit of improving insulin sensitivity, which can help prevent further fat buildup in the liver. Ideally, a combination of cardiovascular and strength training exercises, alongside flexibility practices, should be incorporated into your routine. This combination helps maintain a healthy weight and reduces the fat stored in the liver.

- Regular Screenings: Regular medical screenings are essential for monitoring liver health. Liver function tests and imaging tests, such as ultrasound or fibroscan, can help assess the level of liver damage. In the early stages of fatty liver disease, there may be no symptoms, so it is vital to catch the condition before it progresses to more severe stages. Blood tests, including liver enzymes, can give valuable insight into liver function and help track the progress of the disease. Early diagnosis and intervention increase the chances of successfully reversing fatty liver disease.

By adopting these strategies—dietary improvements, consistent exercise, and routine medical check-ups—individuals in the early stages of fatty liver disease can see significant improvements in liver health. It's essential to make these changes part of your long-term lifestyle, as maintaining liver health requires ongoing commitment.

## Cirrhosis and Beyond

What happens if fatty liver disease progresses to cirrhosis, or if the liver damage becomes too extensive to reverse? This is a question that many facing fatty liver disease may ask as they worry about the future. Unfortunately, once fatty liver disease progresses to cirrhosis, the liver's ability to regenerate becomes much more limited. Cirrhosis is characterized by scarring of the liver tissue, which impairs liver function and makes it difficult for the liver to heal.

While cirrhosis cannot be fully reversed, early intervention and lifestyle changes can still help manage the condition and prevent further damage. In some cases, if the liver is not too severely damaged, the progression of cirrhosis can be halted, and the individual can live a relatively normal life. However, in more severe cases of cirrhosis, the liver may fail, requiring a liver transplant.

The good news is that lifestyle changes still play a significant role, even in these later stages. People with cirrhosis should focus on maintaining a nutritious, liver-friendly diet, staying physically active (within limits), and avoiding substances that may harm the liver further, such as alcohol or drugs. Regular check-ups with a healthcare provider are crucial to monitor the condition and ensure that complications, such as liver cancer or portal hypertension, are prevented or treated early.

The liver's ability to regenerate diminishes as cirrhosis progresses, but early detection, lifestyle modifications, and medical intervention can help manage and control the disease, providing a higher quality of life for those affected. The journey to liver health is not over once fatty liver progresses—it just requires more careful management and attention.

# CHAPTER 12

## Preventing Fatty Liver Disease

When it comes to health, the old saying "Prevention is better than cure" rings truer than ever, especially when it comes to fatty liver disease. With the rising prevalence of non-alcoholic fatty liver disease (NAFLD) globally, it's essential to recognize the signs and act early. After all, prevention offers the best chance to avoid the painful and life-altering consequences of advanced liver disease, such as cirrhosis or liver failure. But the good news is that with the right lifestyle changes, fatty liver disease can be prevented before it even starts.

### Prevention is Better Than Cure

The most powerful tool in preventing fatty liver disease is awareness. Understanding the role of diet, exercise, and stress management is crucial in keeping the liver healthy. By making these foundational lifestyle changes early, you can stop fatty liver disease in its tracks before it ever becomes a problem.

The key to prevention starts with the recognition of risk factors. Conditions such as obesity, type 2 diabetes, high blood pressure, high cholesterol, and insulin resistance are major contributors to fatty liver disease. The sooner you recognize these risk factors and make lifestyle adjustments, the more likely you are to protect your liver from developing fatty liver disease.

Prevention begins with making simple, sustainable changes that you can stick to for life. Rather than drastic overhauls that might only work short-term, it's important to focus on gradual, achievable goals. By eating a balanced diet, staying physically active, and managing stress, you can significantly reduce your risk of fatty liver disease. These changes may seem small at first, but their impact on liver health can be monumental.

## Adopting a Holistic Approach

Preventing fatty liver disease isn't about following a one-size-fits-all plan. It's about adopting a holistic approach that addresses all aspects of your health. This means combining the right diet, regular exercise, and effective stress management techniques to create a well-rounded plan that supports your liver and overall health.

- Diet: A healthy, nutrient-dense diet is foundational in liver health. The liver thrives when it receives an abundance of antioxidants, healthy fats, lean proteins, and fiber. Focus on whole, unprocessed foods like vegetables, fruits, lean meats, whole grains, and healthy fats. Reducing the consumption of sugar, refined carbs, and processed foods helps reduce the strain on your liver and keeps it from accumulating fat.

- Exercise: Consistent physical activity is essential for maintaining metabolic health. Whether it's walking, swimming, cycling, or strength training, exercise helps regulate weight, improve insulin sensitivity, and reduce liver fat. Aim for at least 30 minutes of moderate exercise five days a week. Consistency is key, so make sure that exercise becomes a regular part of your routine.
- Stress Management: Chronic stress can take a toll on both your physical and mental well-being, and it's no different for the liver. Stress triggers the release of hormones that can increase inflammation and affect liver function. To prevent this, incorporate stress-reduction techniques like yoga, meditation, or deep breathing exercises into your daily routine. A calm, balanced mind helps support a healthy body, including a healthy liver.

When all three aspects—diet, exercise, and stress management—work together, they create a holistic system that nurtures your liver and ensures long-term health. You'll notice improvements in energy, mood, and overall health, and your liver will thank you by staying healthy and free from fatty liver disease.

**Staying Consistent**

The most important factor in preventing fatty liver disease is consistency. A healthy lifestyle isn't a short-term fix; it's a lifelong commitment. The key to success lies in making healthy habits part of your daily routine. It's not about perfection—it's about consistency. Small, manageable changes, when done consistently, create lasting results.

Start by setting achievable goals for yourself. This could mean eating one extra serving of vegetables a day, walking for 20 minutes after lunch, or taking five minutes each morning for deep breathing exercises. Don't focus on perfection; focus on creating sustainable habits that become part of your everyday life.

As you begin to see the benefits of your healthy changes—more energy, better sleep, improved mood—you'll be motivated to stick with it. Over time, these habits will become second nature, and you'll no longer have to think about them. They'll just be part of your lifestyle, protecting not only your liver but your overall health.

Remember, prevention doesn't require drastic changes or extreme measures—it requires small, consistent steps that you can incorporate into your daily routine. The good news is that it's never too early to start, and it's never too late to improve your liver health. By making these changes today, you're ensuring that your liver stays strong and healthy for years to come.

# CONCLUSION

As we reach the end of this journey through fatty liver disease and liver health, it's important to remember that the road ahead is within your control. While facing a diagnosis of fatty liver disease can feel overwhelming at first, the good news is that with the right approach, you have the power to take charge of your liver health and make significant strides toward recovery.

We've explored how fatty liver disease can sneak up silently, affecting countless individuals without clear symptoms. But we've also seen that early intervention—through diet, exercise, and stress management—can not only prevent the disease from advancing but can also reverse the damage in its early stages. The liver, with its extraordinary ability to regenerate, offers a unique opportunity for healing, provided it receives the care and attention it deserves.

Taking proactive steps is the key to protecting your liver and ensuring its long-term health. By adopting a holistic approach, you can nurture your liver and prevent fatty liver disease from becoming a life-altering condition. This includes choosing the right foods, staying active, and managing stress effectively. These lifestyle changes, when made consistently, can transform your liver health and help you lead a healthier, more vibrant life.

There is hope—fatty liver disease is not a lifelong sentence. It is a condition that can be managed, reversed, and even prevented. The sooner you start taking action, the better the results you will see. And remember, the power of lifestyle changes is far-reaching. It's not just about avoiding a serious liver condition; it's about improving overall health and reducing the risk of other chronic diseases, like heart disease, type 2 diabetes, and cancer. Your liver, after all, is just one part of the intricate system that keeps you functioning optimally.

Every small change you make is a step toward better health. It's easy to get discouraged when trying to make big shifts in your life, but it's important to remember that small, consistent steps lead to big changes. Whether you're starting with a 10-minute walk or swapping out a sugary snack for a healthier alternative, each choice adds up. As you stick to these changes, you'll begin to notice the positive effects not only on your liver but on your energy levels, mental clarity, and overall well-being.

In closing, I want to leave you with one final thought: you have the power to rewrite your health story. Fatty liver disease may have been a silent threat, but now you have the knowledge and tools to fight back. Take charge of your liver health today, and embrace the journey toward a healthier, happier you. The road to recovery isn't always easy, but with persistence and consistency, you can achieve lasting change.

Your liver's future is bright—and it starts with you.